ALZHEIMER'S DIET
COOKBOOK FOR SENIORS

Quick and easy low carb recipes to enhance brain function and fight memory loss

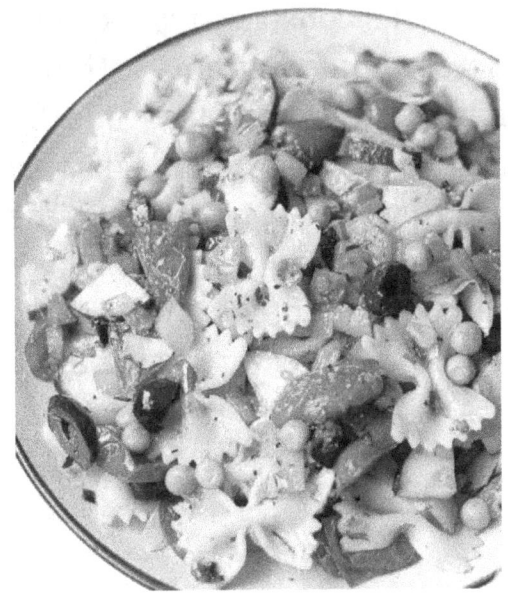

Dr. Malvin Harison

TABLE OF CONTENT

Introduction

Welcome to the Alzheimer's Diet Cookbook for Seniors." In the tapestry of aging, where memories are treasured and the essence of self is delicately woven, the significance of a well-balanced and purposeful diet becomes paramount. This cookbook is not just a collection of recipes; it's a culinary companion designed to support the unique nutritional needs of seniors navigating the challenging terrain of Alzheimer's.

Within these pages, you will discover a symphony of flavors carefully orchestrated to stimulate the senses and nourish the brain.
Each recipe is a testament to the belief that wholesome, thoughtfully chosen ingredients can be a source of joy and vitality, fostering both physical well-being and cognitive resilience.

As we embark on this gastronomic journey, let the aroma of sizzling herbs and the colors of vibrant produce awaken not only the appetite but also a renewed appreciation for the profound connection between the foods we savor and the well-being we cultivate.

Understanding Alzheimer's diet

A Journey through the Alzheimer's Diet." In the intricate dance between nutrition and cognitive well-being, this book unravels the secrets of an Alzheimer's diet. We delve into the art of choosing ingredients that not only nourish the body but also support cognitive health. Let this guide be your compass, navigating the terrain of foods that fuel both body and mind. Join us in understanding the symphony of flavors that harmonize with memory, offering a unique perspective on the Alzheimer's diet—a key to unlocking the potential for a more mindful and vibrant life.

The importance of diet for seniors with Alzheimer's

In the twilight years, when memories are cherished treasures, the importance of a diet cookbook for seniors facing Alzheimer's cannot be overstated.

This cookbook serves as a beacon, illuminating a path towards not just sustenance but a meaningful and nourishing relationship with food.

The essence lies in understanding that every ingredient holds the potential to become a source of comfort, joy, and, most importantly, cognitive support. Carefully curated recipes within these pages are more than a collection of instructions; they are a roadmap for crafting meals that resonate with the unique nutritional needs of seniors grappling with Alzheimer's.

Through mindful nourishment, we aim to provide more than sustenance; we offer a tangible way to enhance the quality of life. Each recipe is a testament to the belief that a well-balanced and purposeful diet can be a source of resilience, promoting both physical well-being and cognitive vitality.

This cookbook is not just about what's on the plate; it's about the memories made around the table, the joy found in a shared meal, and the hope embedded in each bite. It's a culinary companion on the journey of aging,
providing not just recipes but a bridge between the pleasure of eating and the art of nurturing both body and mind.

Complications of not taken the Right Diet

In the context of Alzheimer's disease, not adhering to the right diet can lead to various complications and challenges for seniors. Here are some potential repercussions of not maintaining an appropriate diet:

1. Cognitive Decline: A diet lacking essential nutrients can contribute to cognitive decline, exacerbating the symptoms of Alzheimer's.

Proper nutrition is crucial for supporting brain health and maintaining cognitive function.

2. Weakened Immune System: Inadequate nutrition may compromise the immune system, leaving seniors more susceptible to infections and illnesses. This can lead to additional health complications, impacting overall well-being.

3. Increased Behavioral Issues: Poor nutrition can influence mood and behavior, potentially exacerbating behavioral issues associated with Alzheimer's disease. It may contribute to increased agitation, aggression, or other challenging behaviors.

4. Weight Loss and Malnutrition: Seniors with Alzheimer's often face difficulties in maintaining a healthy weight.

Inadequate nutrition can contribute to weight loss and malnutrition, further diminishing their overall health and resilience.

5. Decreased Quality of Life: A lack of proper nutrients can contribute to a decrease in overall energy levels and vitality, impacting the quality of life for seniors living with Alzheimer's. This can affect their ability to engage in daily activities and enjoy life.

6. Diminished Physical Health: Poor nutrition can have a cascading effect on physical health, leading to complications such as muscle weakness, bone frailty, and a higher risk of falls and fractures.

7. Worsening of Existing Health Conditions: Alzheimer's often coexists with other health conditions. Neglecting the right diet may worsen these coexisting conditions, complicating medical management and overall health outcomes.

8. Increased Caregiver Burden: Inadequate nutrition may necessitate more intensive caregiving, placing an additional burden on caregivers. Ensuring a proper diet can contribute to a more manageable caregiving experience.

Chapter 1: Delicious Breakfast Recipes for Alzheimer's

1. Blueberry Walnut Oatmeal

Ingredients

1. 1/2 cup rolled oats
2. 1 cup blueberries (fresh or frozen)
3. 2 tablespoons chopped walnuts
4. 1 tablespoon honey
5. 1 cup milk (dairy or plant-based)

Instructions

1. Cook oats according to package instructions.
2. Stir in blueberries, walnuts, honey, and milk.
3. Cook for an additional 2-3 minutes until blueberries soften.
4. Serve warm.

Servings: 1

Nutritional Value (per serving)
- Calories: 350
- Fiber
- Omega-3 fatty acids

2. Greek Yogurt Parfait with Berries

Ingredients
1. 1 cup Greek yogurt (low-fat)
2. 1/2 cup mixed berries (strawberries, blueberries, raspberries)
3. 2 tablespoons granola
4. 1 tablespoon chia seeds
5. Drizzle of honey

Instructions
1. In a glass, layer Greek yogurt, mixed berries, granola, and chia seeds.
2. Spray honey on top.
3. Repeat for additional layers.
4. Serve chilled.

Servings: 1

Nutritional Value (per serving)
- Calories: 280
- Protein
- Antioxidants

3. Spinach and Feta Omelette

Ingredients

1. 2 eggs
2. 1/2 cup fresh spinach, chopped
3. 2 tablespoons feta cheese, crumbled
4. 1 tablespoon olive oil
5. Salt and pepper to taste

Instructions

1. Whisk eggs in a bowl.
2. Heat olive oil in a pan and sauté spinach until wilted.
3. Pour whisked eggs over spinach.
4. Sprinkle feta cheese, salt, and pepper.
5. Cook until eggs are set.
6. Fold and serve.

Servings: 1

Nutritional Value (per serving)

- Calories: 320
- Protein
- Vitamin K

4. Avocado Toast with Salmon

Ingredients
1. 1 slice whole-grain bread
2. 1/2 avocado, mashed
3. 2 oz smoked salmon
4. Lemon juice
5. Fresh dill (optional)

Instructions
1. Toast the bread slice.
2. Spread mashed avocado on the toast.
3. Top with smoked salmon.
4. Squeeze lemon juice and garnish with fresh dill if desired.

Servings: 1

Nutritional Value (per serving)
- Calories: 290
- Omega-3 fatty acids
- Fiber

5. Coconut-Berry Smoothie

Ingredients
1. 1/2 cup blueberries
2. 1/2 cup strawberries
3. 1/2 cup raspberries

4. 1/2 cup Greek yogurt (low-fat)

5. 1/2 banana

6. 1 tablespoon chia seeds

Instructions

1. Blend blueberries, strawberries, raspberries, Greek yogurt, banana, and chia seeds until smooth.

2. Pour into a glass and enjoy.

Servings: 1

Nutritional Value (per serving)

- Calories: 150
- Fiber
- Protein

6. Almond Butter Banana Pancakes

Ingredients

1. 1 ripe banana, mashed

2. 2 eggs

3. 2 tablespoons almond butter

4. 1/2 teaspoon baking powder

5. Pinch of cinnamon

Instructions

1. In a bowl, whisk together mashed banana, eggs, almond butter, baking powder, and cinnamon.

2. Heat a non-stick pan and ladle the batter to make pancakes.

3. Cook till bubbles start forming on the surface, then turn and cook the other side.

4. Serve warm.

Servings: 1

Nutritional Value (per serving)

- Calories: 330
- Protein
- Healthy fats

7. Chia Seed Pudding with Mango

Ingredients

1. 3 tablespoons chia seeds
2. 1/2 cup almond milk (unsweetened)
3. 1/2 teaspoon vanilla extract
4. 1/2 mango, diced
5. 1 tablespoon shredded coconut

Instructions

1. Combine chia seeds, almond milk, and vanilla extract in a jar. Keep in the freezer overnight.

2. In the morning, layer chia pudding with diced mango and shredded coconut.

3. Serve chilled.

Servings: 1

Nutritional Value (per serving)

- Calories: 250
- Fiber
- Omega-3 fatty acids

8. Sweet Potato Breakfast Hash

Ingredients

1. 1 small sweet potato, diced
2. 1/4 cup red bell pepper, diced
3. 1/4 cup onion, chopped
4. 1 tablespoon olive oil
5. 2 eggs

Instructions

1. In a skillet, sauté sweet potato, bell pepper, and onion in olive oil until tender.

2. Make a hole in the hash and crack eggs into them.

3. Cover and cook until eggs are done to your liking.

4. Season with salt and pepper.

Servings: 1

Nutritional Value (per serving)

- Calories: 330
- Protein
- Vitamin A

9. Quinoa Fruit Salad

Ingredients

1. 1/2 cup cooked quinoa
2. 1/2 cup mixed berries (blueberries, strawberries, raspberries)
3. 1/2 kiwi, sliced
4. 1 tablespoon honey
5. 1 tablespoon chopped mint

Instructions

1. In a bowl, combine cooked quinoa, mixed berries, and kiwi.
2. Drizzle honey over the fruit salad.
3. Garnish with chopped mint.
4. Toss gently and serve.

Servings: 1

Nutritional Value (per serving)

- Calories: 270
- Fiber

- Antioxidants

10. Cottage Cheese Stuffed Peaches

Ingredients
1. 1 peach, halved and pitted
2. 1/2 cup cottage cheese
3. 1 tablespoon chopped almonds
4. 1 teaspoon honey
5. Sprinkle of cinnamon

Instructions
1. Scoop out a little flesh from each peach half to create a hollow.
2. In a bowl, mix cottage cheese with chopped almonds.
3. Stuff the peach halves with the cottage cheese mixture.
4. Drizzle honey and sprinkle cinnamon on top.

Servings: 1

Nutritional Value (per serving)
- Calories: 230
- Protein
- Calcium

Chapter 2: Nutritious Lunch Recipes for Alzheimer's

Here are 10 delicious, nutrient-rich and easy-to-prepare lunch recipes designed for Alzheimer's management:

1. Salmon and Quinoa Salad

Ingredients
1. 4 oz salmon filet
2. 1/2 cup cooked quinoa
3. 1 cup mixed salad greens
4. 1/4 cup cherry tomatoes, halved
5. Lemon vinaigrette dressing

Instructions
1. Bake salmon until cooked.
2. Arrange salad greens, quinoa, and cherry tomatoes on a plate.
3. Place the cooked salmon on top.
4. Drizzle with lemon vinaigrette dressing.

Servings: 1
Nutritional Value (per serving)
- Calories: 400
- Omega-3 fatty acids
- Protein

2. Chicken and Vegetable Stir-Fry

Ingredients
1. 4 oz chicken breast, sliced
2. 1 cup broccoli florets
3. 1/2 bell pepper, sliced
4. 1/2 cup snap peas
5. 1 tablespoon olive oil
6. Low-sodium soy sauce

Instructions
1. Heat olive oil in a pan, add sliced chicken and cook until browned.
2. Add broccoli, bell pepper, and snap peas. Stir-fry until vegetables are tender.
3. Drizzle with low-sodium soy sauce.

Servings: 1
Nutritional Value (per serving)
- Calories: 350
- Protein
- Fiber

3. Turkey and Spinach Stuffed Sweet Potatoes

Ingredients

1. 1 medium sweet potato
2. 4 oz ground turkey
3. 1 cup fresh spinach
4. 1/4 cup feta cheese, crumbled
5. Olive oil for drizzling

Instructions

1. Bake sweet potatoes until tender.
2. In a pan, cook ground turkey until browned.
3. Add fresh spinach to the pan and cook until wilted.
4. Split the sweet potato and fill with the turkey and spinach mixture.
5. Top with crumbled feta and drizzle with olive oil.

Servings: 1

Nutritional Value (per serving)

- Calories: 380
- Protein
- Vitamin A

4. Vegetarian Quinoa Bowl

Ingredients
1. 1/2 cup cooked quinoa
2. 1/2 cup chickpeas (canned, drained)
3. 1/2 cup cucumber, diced
4. 1/4 cup feta cheese, crumbled
5. Kalamata olives, sliced
6. Hummus for dressing

Instructions
1. Arrange quinoa, chickpeas, cucumber, feta, and olives in a bowl.
2. Spray with hummus for dressing.

Servings: 1

Nutritional Value (per serving)
- Calories: 320
- Protein
- Fiber

5. Lentil and Vegetable Soup

Ingredients
1. 1/2 cup dry lentils
2. 1 cup mixed vegetables (carrots, celery, onions)
3. 2 cups low-sodium vegetable broth

4. 1 teaspoon olive oil

5. Herbs and spices to taste (thyme, rosemary)

Instructions

1. Rinse lentils and cook in vegetable broth until tender.

2. Sauté mixed vegetables in olive oil until soft.

3. Combine lentils, vegetables, and herbs.

Servings: 1

Nutritional Value (per serving)

- Calories: 280
- Protein
- Fiber

6. Mediterranean Tuna Salad Wrap

Ingredients

1. 1 whole-grain wrap
2. 1/2 cup canned tuna, drained
3. 1/4 cup cherry tomatoes, halved
4. 2 tablespoons black olives, sliced
5. 1 tablespoon olive oil
6. Mixed greens

Instructions

1. Mix tuna, cherry tomatoes, and black olives.
2. Lay out a whole-grain wrap and add the tuna mixture.
3. Drizzle with olive oil and add mixed greens.
4. Roll into a wrap.

Servings: 1

Nutritional Value (per serving)

- Calories: 340
- Omega-3 fatty acids
- Protein

7. Shrimp and Broccoli Quinoa Bowl

Ingredients

1. 4 oz shrimp, peeled and deveined
2. 1 cup broccoli florets
3. 1/2 cup cooked quinoa
4. 1 tablespoon sesame oil
5. Low-sodium soy sauce

Instructions

1. Sauté shrimp in sesame oil until cooked.
2. Steam broccoli until tender.

3. Combine shrimp, broccoli, and quinoa in a bowl.

4. Drizzle with low-sodium soy sauce.

Servings: 1

Nutritional Value (per serving)

- Calories: 320
- Protein
- Fiber

8. Egg and Vegetable Wrap

Ingredients

1. 2 eggs, beaten
2. 1 whole-grain wrap
3. 1/2 cup bell peppers, diced
4. 1/4 cup red onion, diced
5. 1 tablespoon olive oil

Instructions

1. Sauté bell peppers and red onion in olive oil.

2. Pour beaten eggs into the pan and scramble.

3. Lay out a whole-grain wrap and add the egg and vegetable mixture.

4. Roll into a wrap.

Servings: 1

Nutritional Value (per serving)
- Calories: 310
- Protein
- Vitamin C

9. Chickpea and Avocado Salad

Ingredients
1. 1/2 cup canned chickpeas, drained
2. 1/2 avocado, diced
3. 1/4 cup cucumber, diced
4. Cherry tomatoes, halved
5. Lemon-tahini dressing

Instructions
1. Combine chickpeas, avocado, cucumber, and cherry tomatoes in a bowl.
2. Drizzle with lemon-tahini dressing.

Servings: 1

Nutritional Value (per serving)
- Calories: 360
- Protein
- Healthy fats

10. Roasted Vegetable Quiche

Ingredients

1. 1 whole-grain pie crust
2. 4 eggs, beaten
3. 1/2 cup milk (dairy or plant-based)
4. 1 cup mixed roasted vegetables (zucchini, bell peppers, tomatoes)
5. 1/4 cup feta cheese, crumbled

Instructions

1. Preheat the oven and blind-bake the pie crust.
2. Whisk eggs and milk in a bowl.
3. Layer roasted vegetables and feta in the pie crust.
4. Pour the egg mixture over the vegetables.
5. Bake until the quiche is set.

Servings: 4 (for a pie)

Nutritional Value (per serving)

- Calories: 280
- Protein
- Vitamin A

Chapter 3: Satisfying Dinner Recipes for Alzheimer's

Here are 10 delicious, nutrient-rich, and easy-to-prepare dinner recipes tailored for Alzheimer's management:

1. Baked Lemon Garlic Salmon

Ingredients
1. 4 oz salmon filet
2. 1 tablespoon olive oil
3. 1 lemon, sliced
4. 2 cloves garlic, minced
5. Fresh dill for garnish

Instructions
1. Preheat the oven to 375°F (190°C).
2. Place salmon on a baking sheet.
3. Drizzle with olive oil, sprinkle minced garlic, and lay lemon slices on top.
4. Bake for 15-20 minutes until the salmon is cooked.

5. Garnish with fresh dill before serving.
Servings: 1
Nutritional Value (per serving)
- Calories: 350
- Omega-3 fatty acids
- Protein

2. Quinoa and Vegetable Stir-Fry

Ingredients
1. 1/2 cup cooked quinoa
2. 1 cup mixed vegetables (broccoli, bell peppers, carrots)
3. 4 oz tofu, cubed
4. 1 tablespoon soy sauce (low-sodium)
5. 1 teaspoon sesame oil

Instructions
1. Sauté tofu in sesame oil until golden.
2. Add mixed vegetables and cook until tender.
3. Stir in cooked quinoa and soy sauce.
4. Cook for an additional 2-3 minutes.
5. Serve hot.

Servings: 1
Nutritional Value (per serving)
- Calories: 320

- Protein
- Fiber

3. Mushroom and Spinach Stuffed Chicken Breast

Ingredients
1. 1 boneless, skinless chicken breast
2. 1/2 cup mushrooms, chopped
3. 1 cup fresh spinach
4. 2 tablespoons feta cheese, crumbled
5. 1 tablespoon olive oil

Instructions
1. Preheat the oven to 400°F (200°C).
2. Butterfly the chicken breast.
3. Sauté mushrooms and spinach in olive oil until wilted.
4. Stuff the chicken breast with the mushroom and spinach mixture.
5. Bake for at least 25-30 minutes till the chicken is cooked.
6. Sprinkle with feta before serving.
Servings: 1

Nutritional Value (per serving)
- Calories: 380

- Protein
- Vitamin D

4. Cauliflower and Chickpea Curry

Ingredients
1. 1 cup cauliflower florets
2. 1/2 cup canned chickpeas, drained
3. 1/2 cup tomatoes, diced
4. 1/2 cup coconut milk (unsweetened)
5. 1 tablespoon curry powder

Instructions
1. In a pan, sauté cauliflower, chickpeas, and tomatoes.
2. Add curry powder and stir.
3. Pour in coconut milk and simmer until cauliflower is tender.
4. Serve over brown rice.

Servings: 1

Nutritional Value (per serving)
- Calories: 340
- Fiber
- Plant-based protein

5. Grilled Turkey and Vegetable Kebabs

Ingredients

1. 4 oz turkey breast, cut into cubes
2. Bell peppers, cherry tomatoes, zucchini (vegetables of choice)
3. Olive oil
4. Garlic powder
5. Italian seasoning

Instructions

1. Preheat the grill.
2. Thread turkey and vegetables onto skewers.
3. Drizzle with olive oil and sprinkle with garlic powder and Italian seasoning.
4. Grill until turkey is cooked and vegetables are charred.
5. Serve hot.

Servings: 1

Nutritional Value (per serving)

- Calories: 320
- Protein
- Vitamin C

6. Sweet Potato and Black Bean Chili

Ingredients

1. 1 cup sweet potatoes, diced
2. 1/2 cup black beans (canned, drained)
3. 1/2 cup tomatoes, diced
4. 1/2 cup corn kernels
5. Chili powder and cumin to taste

Instructions

1. In a pot, combine sweet potatoes, black beans, tomatoes, and corn.
2. Add chili powder and cumin to taste.
3. Simmer until sweet potatoes are tender.
4. Serve with a dollop of Greek yogurt.

Servings: 1

Nutritional Value (per serving)

- Calories: 330
- Fiber
- Antioxidants

7. Eggplant and Tomato Stew

Ingredients

1. 1 small eggplant, diced
2. 1 cup tomatoes, diced

3. 1/2 cup chickpeas (canned, drained)

4. 1/4 cup olives, sliced

5. Fresh basil for garnish

Instructions

1. Sauté eggplant until golden.

2. Add tomatoes, chickpeas, and olives. Cook until vegetables are tender.

3. Garnish with fresh basil before serving.

4. Serve over quinoa.

Servings: 1

Nutritional Value (per serving)

- Calories: 310

- Fiber

- Plant-based protein

8. Salmon and Asparagus Foil Packets

Ingredients

1. 4 oz salmon filet

2. Asparagus spears

3. Lemon slices

4. Dill and garlic for seasoning

5. Olive oil

Instructions

1. Preheat the oven to 400°F (200°C).

2. Place salmon on a piece of foil.

3. Arrange asparagus around the salmon.

4. Drizzle with olive oil, sprinkle dill and garlic.

5. Seal the foil packet and bake for 15-20 minutes.

6. Serve hot.

Servings: 1

Nutritional Value (per serving)

- Calories: 360
- Omega-3 fatty acids
- Protein

9. Vegetable and Quinoa Stuffed Bell Peppers

Ingredients

1. 2 bell peppers, halved and seeds removed

2. 1/2 cup cooked quinoa

3. 1/2 cup black beans (canned, drained)

4. 1/2 cup corn kernels

5. Salsa for topping

Instructions

1. Preheat the oven to 375°F (190°C).
2. In a bowl, mix quinoa, black beans, and corn.
3. Stuff bell peppers with the quinoa mixture.
4. Bake for 25-30 minutes until peppers are tender.
5. Top with salsa before serving.

Servings: 1

Nutritional Value (per serving)

- Calories: 340
- Fiber
- Plant-based protein

10. Chicken and Broccoli Brown Rice Bowl

Ingredients

1. 4 oz chicken breast, cooked and shredded
2. 1 cup broccoli florets
3. 1/2 cup brown rice, cooked
4. 1 tablespoon soy sauce (low-sodium)
5. Sesame seeds for garnish

Instructions

1. Sauté broccoli in a pan until tender.

2. Add shredded chicken, cooked brown rice, and soy sauce.

3. Stir until well combined.

4. Garnish with sesame seeds before serving.

Servings: 1

Nutritional Value (per serving)

- Calories: 380
- Protein
- Fiber

Chapter 4: Easy-to-prepare Snacks and Dessert

Here are 10 delicious, nutrient-rich snacks and dessert recipes suitable for Alzheimer's management:

1. Nutty Banana Bites

Ingredients
1. 1 banana, sliced
2. 2 tablespoons almond butter
3. Chopped nuts (almonds, walnuts)

Instructions
1. Spread almond butter on banana slices.
2. Sprinkle with chopped nuts.
3. Serve immediately.

Servings: 1

Nutritional Value (per serving)
- Calories: 180
- Healthy fats

- Potassium

2. Greek Yogurt Parfait with Berries

Ingredients
1. 1/2 cup Greek yogurt (low-fat)
2. 1/4 cup mixed berries (blueberries, strawberries)
3. 2 tablespoons granola
4. Drizzle of honey

Instructions
1. Layer Greek yogurt, berries, and granola.
2. Drizzle with honey.
3. Repeat for additional layers.
4. Serve chilled.

Servings: 1

Nutritional Value (per serving)
- Calories: 200
- Protein
- Antioxidants

3. Dark Chocolate Avocado Mousse

Ingredients

1. 1 ripe avocado
2. 2 tablespoons cocoa powder (unsweetened)
3. 2 tablespoons maple syrup
4. 1/2 teaspoon vanilla extract

Instructions

1. Blend avocado until smooth.
2. Combine cocoa powder, maple syrup, and vanilla extract.
3. Blend until creamy.
4. Refrigerate before serving.

Servings: 2

Nutritional Value (per serving)

- Calories: 150
- Healthy fats
- Antioxidants

4. Cinnamon Apple Slices

Ingredients

1. 1 apple, sliced
2. 1 tablespoon almond butter
3. Sprinkle of cinnamon

Instructions

1. Spread almond butter on apple slices.
2. Sprinkle with cinnamon.
3. Serve immediately.

Servings: 1

Nutritional Value (per serving)

- Calories: 120
- Fiber
- Vitamin C

5. Frozen Berry Yogurt Bites

Ingredients

1. 1 cup Greek yogurt (low-fat)
2. 1/2 cup mixed berries (blueberries, raspberries)
3. 1 tablespoon honey

Instructions

1. Mix Greek yogurt, berries, and honey.
2. Spoon into small silicone molds.
3. Freeze until solid.
4. Pop out and enjoy.

Servings: 4

Nutritional Value (per serving)

- Calories: 50
- Protein

- Antioxidants

6. Chia Seed Pudding with Mango

Ingredients
1. 3 tablespoons chia seeds
2. 1/2 cup almond milk (unsweetened)
3. 1/2 teaspoon vanilla extract
4. 1/2 mango, diced
5. 1 tablespoon shredded coconut

Instructions
1. Mingle chia seeds, almond milk, and vanilla extract in a jar. Keep in freezer overnight.
2. In the morning, layer chia pudding with diced mango and shredded coconut.
3. Serve chilled.

Servings: 1

Nutritional Value (per serving)
- Calories: 250
- Fiber
- Omega-3 fatty acids

7. Baked Cinnamon Banana Chips

Ingredients
1. 2 bananas, sliced
2. 1 tablespoon coconut oil (melted)
3. 1 teaspoon cinnamon

Instructions
1. Preheat the oven to 200°F (93°C).
2. Toss banana slices in melted coconut oil and cinnamon.
3. Arrange on a baking sheet and bake for 2-3 hours.
4. Let cool before serving.

Servings: 2

Nutritional Value (per serving)
- Calories: 90
- Potassium
- Natural sugars

8. Coconut Almond Energy Bites

Ingredients
1. 1/2 cup almonds, finely chopped
2. 1/2 cup shredded coconut (unsweetened)
3. 2 tablespoons coconut oil (melted)

4. 1 tablespoon honey

5. 1/2 teaspoon vanilla extract

Instructions

1. Mix chopped almonds, shredded coconut, melted coconut oil, honey, and vanilla extract in a bowl.

2. Form into bite-sized balls.

3. Refrigerate until firm.

Servings: 8

Nutritional Value (per serving)

- Calories: 90

- Healthy fats

- Protein

9. Berry and Spinach Smoothie

Ingredients

1. 1/2 cup mixed berries (blueberries, strawberries)

2. 1/2 banana

3. Handful of spinach leaves

4. 1/2 cup Greek yogurt (low-fat)

5. 1/2 cup water

Instructions

1. Blend berries, banana, spinach, Greek yogurt, and water until smooth.

2. Pour into a glass and enjoy.

Servings: 1

Nutritional Value (per serving)

- Calories: 150
- Fiber
- Vitamin K

10. Almond Butter and Banana Oat Cookies

Ingredients

1. 1 cup rolled oats
2. 1/2 cup almond butter
3. 1 ripe banana, mashed
4. 1/2 teaspoon vanilla extract
5. 1/4 cup dark chocolate chips (optional)

Instructions

1. Preheat the oven to 350°F (175°C).
2. Mix rolled oats, almond butter, mashed banana, vanilla extract, and dark chocolate chips.
3. Spoon onto a baking sheet and flatten.
4. Bake for 12-15 minutes until golden.

Servings: 12

Nutritional Value (per serving)

- Calories: 80
- Fiber
- Healthy fats

Bonus: 20 Juicing and Smoothie Recipes for Alzheimer's Management

1. Green Brain Boost

Ingredients
1. 1 cup kale
2. 1/2 cucumber
3. 1 green apple
4. 1/2 lemon (peeled)
5. 1-inch ginger

Instructions
1. Wash and chop ingredients.
2. Juice and enjoy immediately.

2. Berry Bliss

Ingredients
1. 1 cup blueberries
2. 1 cup strawberries
3. 1/2 cup blackberries
4. 1/2 cup Greek yogurt (low-fat)
5. 1/2 cup water

Instructions

1. Rinse berries.
2. Blend all ingredients until smooth.

3. Citrus Symphony

Ingredients

1. 2 oranges (peeled)
2. 1 grapefruit (peeled)
3. 1 lime (peeled)
4. 1/2 cup pineapple chunks

Instructions

1. Peel and segment citrus fruits.
2. Juice and serve chilled.

4. Carrot and Turmeric Elixir

Ingredients

1. 4 large carrots
2. 1 orange (peeled)
3. 1-inch turmeric root

Instructions

1. Wash and peel carrots.
2. Juice carrots, orange, and turmeric.

5. Beetroot Power Punch

Ingredients

1. 1 beetroot (peeled)
2. 1 apple
3. 1/2 cup raspberries
4. 1 tablespoon chia seeds

Instructions

1. Wash and chop ingredients.
2. Juice and stir in chia seeds.

6. Mango Avocado Bliss

Ingredients

1. 1 cup mango chunks
2. 1/2 avocado
3. 1/2 cup spinach leaves
4. 1/2 cup coconut water

Instructions

1. Blend all ingredients until creamy.

7. Pineapple Ginger Zing

Ingredients

1. 1 cup pineapple chunks
2. 1/2 banana

3. 1/2 teaspoon fresh ginger (grated)
4. 1/2 cup almond milk
Instructions
1. Blend pineapple, banana, ginger, and almond milk.

8. Blueberry Almond Delight

Ingredients
1. 1 cup blueberries
2. 1/2 cup Greek yogurt (low-fat)
3. 1/4 cup almonds
4. 1/2 cup water
Instructions
1. Blend all ingredients until smooth.

9. Spinach and Berry Burst

Ingredients
1. 1 cup spinach leaves
2. 1/2 cup strawberries
3. 1/2 cup raspberries
4. 1/2 cup coconut water
Instructions
1. Rinse berries and spinach.

2. Blend with coconut water until creamy.

10. Turmeric Mango Tango

Ingredients
1. 1 cup mango chunks
2. 1/2 teaspoon turmeric powder
3. 1/2 cup orange juice
4. 1/2 cup water

Instructions
1. Blend mango, turmeric, orange juice, and water until smooth.

11. Spinach Apple Detox

Ingredients
1. 2 cups spinach leaves
2. 2 green apples
3. 1/2 cucumber
4. 1/2 lemon (peeled)

Instructions
1. Wash and chop ingredients.
2. Juice spinach, apples, cucumber, and lemon.
3. Pour into a glass and enjoy.

12. Minty Watermelon Refresher

Ingredients

1. 2 cups watermelon chunks
2. 1/2 cup fresh mint leaves
3. 1 lime (peeled)
4. 1/2 cup strawberries

Instructions

1. Rinse strawberries and mint.
2. Juice watermelon, mint, lime, and strawberries.
3. Serve over ice.

13. Orange Carrot Ginger Elixir

Ingredients

1. 4 large carrots
2. 3 oranges (peeled)
3. 1-inch ginger

Instructions

1. Wash and peel carrots.
2. Juice carrots, oranges, and ginger.
3. Pour into a glass and enjoy.

14. Pineapple Kale Twist

Ingredients
1. 1 cup pineapple chunks
2. 2 cups kale leaves
3. 1/2 cucumber
4. 1/2 lemon (peeled)

Instructions
1. Wash and chop ingredients.
2. Juice pineapple, kale, cucumber, and lemon.
3. Stir and serve.

15. Berry Citrus Fusion

Ingredients
1. 1 cup mixed berries (blueberries, raspberries)
2. 2 oranges (peeled)
3. 1/2 grapefruit (peeled)
4. 1/2 cup blackberries

Instructions
1. Rinse berries.
2. Juice oranges, grapefruit, and berries.
3. Pour into a glass and enjoy.

16. Cocoa Banana Bliss

Ingredients
1. 1 banana
2. 1 tablespoon cocoa powder (unsweetened)
3. 1/2 cup almond milk
4. 1 tablespoon almond butter

Instructions
1. Blend banana, cocoa powder, almond milk, and almond butter until smooth.

17. Kiwi Pineapple Pleasure

Ingredients
1. 2 kiwis (peeled)
2. 1 cup pineapple chunks
3. 1/2 cup spinach leaves
4. 1/2 cup coconut water

Instructions
1. Blend kiwis, pineapple, spinach, and coconut water until creamy.

18. Raspberry Almond Dream

Ingredients

1. 1 cup raspberries
2. 1/2 cup almond milk
3. 1/4 cup almonds
4. 1 tablespoon chia seeds

Instructions

1. Blend raspberries, almond milk, almonds, and chia seeds until well mixed.

19. Strawberry Basil Refresher

Ingredients

1. 1 cup strawberries
2. 1/2 cup fresh basil leaves
3. 1/2 cup Greek yogurt (low-fat)
4. 1/2 cup water

Instructions

1. Rinse strawberries and basil.
2. Blend with Greek yogurt and water until smooth.

20. Papaya Coconut Smoothie

Ingredients
1. 1 cup papaya chunks
2. 1/2 cup coconut milk
3. 1/2 banana
4. 1 tablespoon flax seeds

Instructions
1. Blend papaya, coconut milk, banana, and flaxseeds until creamy.

These refreshing juices are packed with nutrients and are a delicious way to support brain health. Enjoy!

BONUS 2: 14 WEEKS
MEAL PLANNER

Conclusion

The journey to managing Alzheimer's through thoughtful nutrition is a path paved with delicious and nutritious choices. The recipes provided not only tantalize the taste buds but also prioritize the well-being of the mind. Incorporating these nutrient-rich meals, snacks, and beverages into your routine can be a positive step towards supporting cognitive health.

Remember, every bite and sip can be a celebration of nourishment for both body and mind. May these recipes bring not only sustenance but also joy to your culinary exploration on the road to Alzheimer's management. Embrace the power of wholesome ingredients, savor the flavors, and cherish the well-being they bring.